About the author:

Fredrick Artis has been involved in fitness and martial arts for the last 30 years. He is a certified nutritionist as well as a certified self-defense instructor. He has been a personal trainer to a multitude of students, men women as well as children. Fredrick has the experience and passion to help his students expand their abilities. His innovative techniques and robust determination makes for the perfect recipe, as a health and fitness advisor.

'About the Book'

This book was written so that anyone can learn to eat well and be healthy. It provides the reader with many recipes that are both healthy
and delicious. With an emphasis on reliable weight loss.

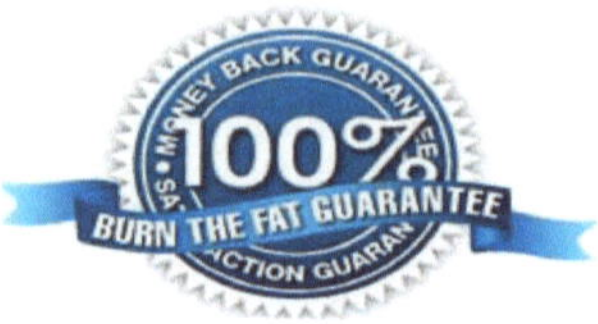

THE PLAN

Eat right, lose weight, live longer. The first key to your plan, would be Not to starve yourself. STARVATION IS BAD. Your body is an amazing Machine, when you dramatically reduce your food intake your brain Responds by lowering the body's metabolism allowing the body to store more fat. Subsequently your body will begin to break down muscle for energy. Therefore, you should eat no less than four to six reasonably size Meals per day. Drink no less than six to eight glasses of water per day. Your body remains at a constant 98 degrees, so if you were to drink an ice cold glass of water. Your body would respond by raising its metabolism to maintain your body temperature. Doing so will burn calories. Eight cups of ice cold water can burn up to 100 calories in a day. Many foods can be harmful to the body, but many can be a great nutritional value as well. In this program you will be given a list of foods that work best with the fat burning process. This will be your main resource for your weight loss. You may eat anything on the list in any combination. However if it is not on the list then you must not eat it during this program

THINGS TO KNOW ABOUT WEIGHT LOSS & HEALTH

Although starvation is bad, lowering your calorie intake is very good. About 72% of Americans are overweight! Now it's time to make a change. Did you know that a low calorie diet can increase your life span? Cheolkoo Lee, a researcher in the Environmental Toxicology Center at the University of Wisconsin in Madison. Found that aging, activates several genes in the brain that causes inflammation. This process damages vital brain cells to the point where they eventually fail. Decreasing calorie intake by 25% suppresses this gene thereby Creating a longer life span.

It can take up to 20min for the stomach to signal the brain that it is full. Therefore if you stop eating when you feel close to being full. Just wait Twenty minutes and perhaps you will find that you truly are full. Visceral fat, also known as organ fat, is located inside the peritoneal Cavity, packed in between internal organs, as opposed to subcutaneous fat which is found underneath the skin an excess of visceral fat leads to the "pot belly" or "beer belly" effect, in which the abdomen protrudes excessively. This body type is also known as "apple" shaped, as opposed to "pear" shape, in which fat is deposited on the hips and buttocks. Visceral fat accumulation is associated with insulin resistance, glucose intolerance, hypertension, and coronary artery disease. Belly fat can be a health danger, typically if a man's waist measures more than 40 inches and a woman's measures grater that 35 inches than this can be associated with having excess visceral fat.

DID YOU KNOW

People with large bellies tend to lose sensitivity to insulin, a crucial Hormone that helps the body burn energy. When insulin loses its power, the body responds by pumping out more of the hormone, which only throws the system further off balance

THE WAY IT IS

It's not hard to find out if you have a potentially unhealthy amount of Belly fat. All you need is a tape measure. Exhale, relax, and wrap the Measure around your stomach. The bottom of the tape should be exactly even with the top of your hip bone. Keep the tape straight and snug, but don't let it dig into your skin. If you're a man, a waist circumference of less than 100 cm (39 inches) means you're unlikely to have trouble with insulin resistance. Women can probably rest easy if their waist is less than 88 cm (34.5 inches) around. Anything above these figures, however, may put you at a higher risk.

Let's start out with some important information on weight loss a technique called "Intermittent fasting"

Intermittent fasting is a beneficial tactic resulting in fat loss and muscle gain. Intermittent fasting

Do not confuse intermittent fasting with dieting because to put in plain terms it isn't a diet at all. It's a scheduled set of eating patterns. Intermittent fasting doesn't focus on what you eat it is more so attributed to when you eat. The logic behind this is extremely interesting, and leaves out the rigorous difficulties of tedious dieting and calorie cutting. Intermittent fasting will also help keep your lean muscle while burning excess unwanted stubborn fat thereby creating that desirable healthy and lean look. Essentially this can allow you to lose fat without any extrema changes in your eating choices.

Here is how Intermittent fasting works.

Let's break this up into two states, called your Fed state and your Fasted state. When your body is digesting and absorbing food this is known as your Fed state. This state extends out from the time you begin eating and throughout your digesting period which usually last around 5 hours. During your fed state your insulin levels increases thereby making it more difficult for your body to burn fat. Once your body is past this state it evolves into what's known as a post-absorptive state. This is the state when your body is no longer absorbing food. This state ranges between 8-12 hours after your last meal and is called your Fasted state. During your Fasted state your insulin levels are low because your body does not need to digest food allowing you to burn more body fat.

When you're in the fasted state your body can burn fat that has been inaccessible during the fed state. It generally takes about 12 hours after your last meal before you enter a Fasted state this is known as your bodies' fat burning state. Think about it when exercising in this stated (Fasted state) your body has no food in its stomach causing it to begin burning stored fat immediately.

Long-term fasting or low calorie diets may not have the same benefits provided by intermittent fasting as it relates to weight loss. Intermittent fasting enhances your hormone receptors that causes a metabolic change forging your body into a fat burning furnace. This causes your body to consume fat as energy rather than glucose (sugar).

Train your body to burning fat rather than sugar.
Fat is a far more efficient form of energy than sugar as it relates to your body. For instance, you can gain twice as much energy while releasing the same amount of free radicals as you would from sugar In fact if your body is primarily burning sugar as a source of energy it will generally cause you to have higher levels of blood sugar which creates much higher rates of sugar-cross-linking of protein molecules, causing internal and external wrinkling of one's tissues, inflammation and stiffness, and premature aging and a hastened pathway to sickness and death. Sugar is stored mostly in the muscles and the blood stream so it's readily available. In any physical activity the body is trained to always burn sugar for approximately the first 12 minutes. At that 12 minute mark the body then decides whether to keep burning sugar or to switch fuels and to start burning fat.

Your body has memory and can easily adapt to regularity

Therefore your body will become accustomed to its usual regimen. If your body has been burning sugar constantly throughout the day then you can expect it to continue to do so at night even while you are sleeping.

If you eat Fat and sugar together your body begins to burn the sugar first. Sugar can cause damage by glycosylation, basically having it around too long can and also accelerate aging. When your body keeps a hold of the sugar it will need to burn off the majority of that sugar before it will start burning fat.

Eating fat is not the cause of obesity rather it is the lack of determination to get rid of it thereby causing your body to store the remaining fat. We become sugar burners by eating sugar and carbohydrates until our leptin levels go so high that our hypothalamus stops listening to leptin and assumes that we are starving.

What is the Hypothalamus: The **hypothalamus** is a section of the brain responsible for the production of many of the body's essential hormones, chemical substances that help control different cells and organs. The hormones from the hypothalamus govern physiologic functions such as temperature regulation, thirst, hunger, sleep, mood, sex drive, and the release of other hormones within the body. This area of the brain houses the pituitary gland and other glands in the body.

Although this portion of the brain is small in size, it is involved in many necessary processes of the body including behavioral, autonomic (involuntary or unconscious), and endocrine functions, such as metabolism and growth and development.

Sugar burns quickly in the body, this causes much wasted energy from damaging free radicals. The majority of the cells in the body excluding your brain cells are geared to burn strictly sugar for a short duration in times of exigency, when the damage from free radicals is not as important as dealing with the emergency. However our bodies are designed to store fat, although we can also store small amounts of sugar which is then converted into the form of glycogen enough to last for 30 to 40 minutes of extreme exertion.

SECRETS OF THE DIET EXPERTS

Chew your food thoroughly (This gives your brain time to Signal the body that it had enough) Drink at least six glasses of Water every day

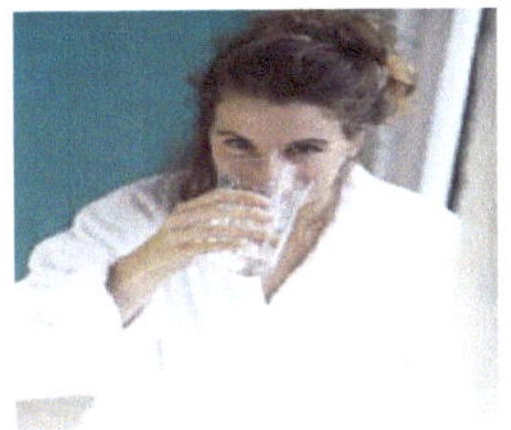

When under stress your body produces cortical.
Cortisol, sometimes called "the stress hormone," is a hormone produced by the adrenal glands that helps regulate blood pressure and cardiovascular Function as well as the metabolism and breakdown of proteins, Carbohydrates and fats. Cortisol secretion increases in response to physical and psychological stress. At normal levels, cortisol helps the body react to stress appropriately and Provides sources of energy; high, prolonged levels of cortisol in the Bloodstream have been shown to have negative effects, such as impaired Cognitive performance, suppressed thyroid function, blood sugar imbalances, Decreased bone density decrease in muscle tissue, higher blood presser and Increased abdominal fat. Spicy foods can raise your metabolism Capsaicin is the active component in chili peppers that Causes a rise in heat generation. Which helps to burn more? Calories immediately after a meal, as do (Ginger & Black Pepper)

Breakdown of Fat Types
In Various Oils

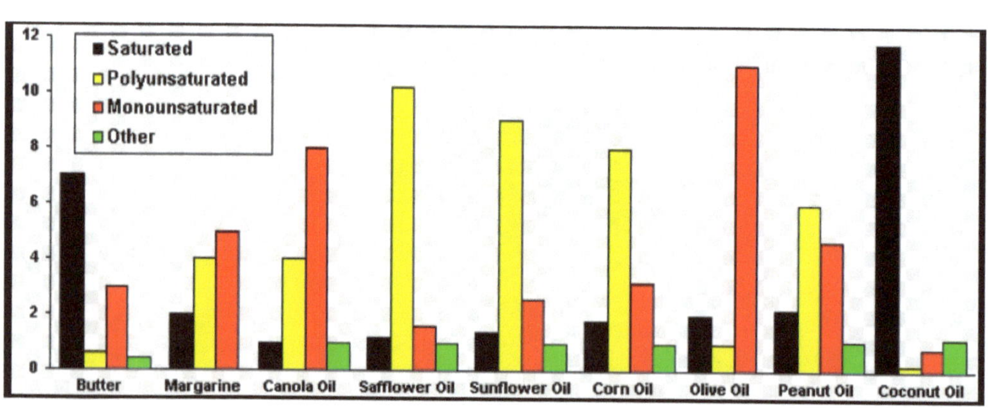

Aren't ALL Fats Bad?

No. There are "good" fats and "bad" ones, just like there's good and Bad blood cholesterol. Saturated fats and Tran's fat have bad effects on cholesterol levels. Polyunsaturated fats and monounsaturated fats (such As olive oil, canola oil, soybean oil, and corn oil) have good effects.

Definitions:

Saturated Fats - Saturated fat and Tran's fat both raise LDL ("bad")

Cholesterol, which increases the risk of developing coronary heart disease.

Monounsaturated Fats - Monounsaturated fats can have a beneficial Effect on your health... when eaten in moderation and when used to replace saturated fats or Trans fats. Monounsaturated fats can help reduce bad cholesterol levels in your blood and lower your risk of heart disease and stroke.

Polyunsaturated Fats - Polyunsaturated fatty acids include the Essential fatty acids, linoleic acid and alpha-linoleic acid. A number of other polyunsaturated fatty acids occur in high concentrations in fish and vegetable oils and are thought to be particularly beneficial to health

Trans Fatty Acid - It's important to know about trans-fat because there is a direct, proven relationship between diets high in trans-fat content and LDL ("bad") Cholesterol levels and, therefore, an increased risk of coronary heart disease – a leading cause of death in the US Trans Fatty Acid is fat manufactured which is worse than saturated fats.

STOP FOOD CRAVINGS

Starvation is usually misunderstood as a quick fix, but this Assumption is absolutely not true. Instead, to burn fat you need To be consistently feeding your body throughout the day with The right foods. You should eat four to six meals using the right Foods. This is the best way to keep your body regulated for Maximum fat burning. You should note that skipping meals Can cause you to splurge latter. So the key would be to eat less And more often. Digestion burns calories, so eat small frequent Meals to keep your inner Furness burning. Are you hungry, are you sure, often hunger can be mistaken for thirst. Therefore drinking many glasses of water during the day can assist in preventing uncontrollable junk food splurges. When dehydrated you become physically and mentally Sluggish and when you are feeling thirsty you are already dehydrated. Think about this. The reason you are being told to eat several small meals a day is because if your body believes it isn't getting enough food. It will go into starvation mode and hold onto every bit of fat that it can.

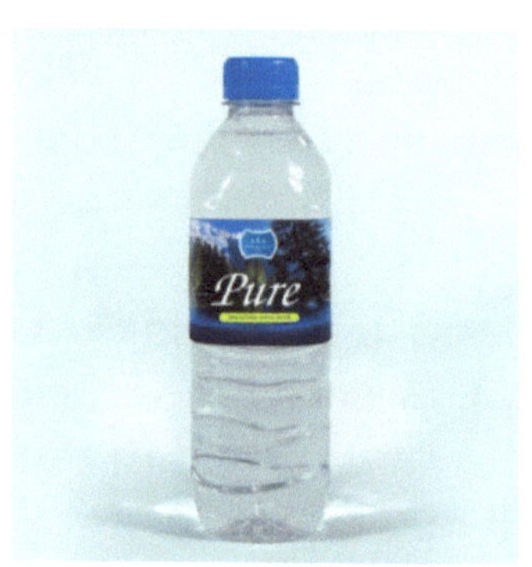

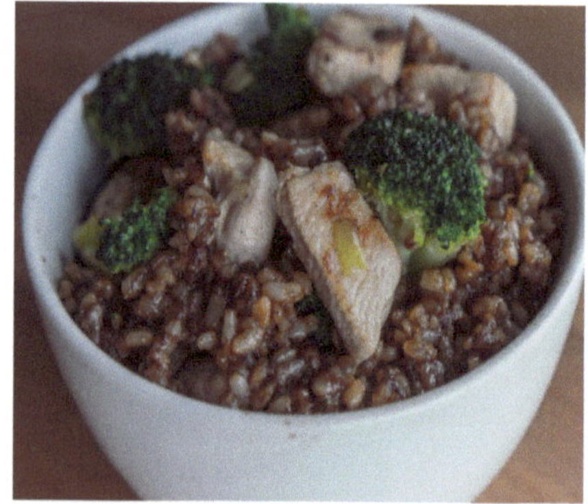

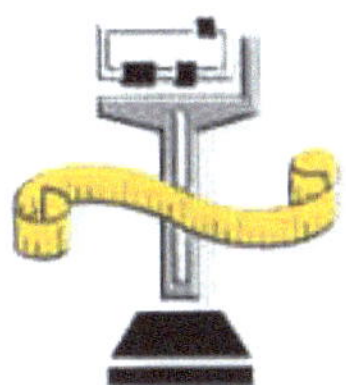

One thing you should know about the human body is that
Losing weight can slow down your metabolism. So as a result,
The more you lose the slower you will continue to lose. So if you
Were to lose a substantial amount of weight in the beginning
But not as much as the program continues. Don't be
Discouraged you are doing just fine

Below is the key to this program, this is your lifeline per say. Here is a list of the foods you can consume during the duration of this three week program. You are able to eat anything on the list in any combination, however if it is not on the list then it cannot be eaten. It's just that simple. Make sure to consume 4 to 6 small meals per day and observe the weight melt away. Also drink no less than 8 glasses of water daily for optimum results.

(THE LIST)

BEANS
GREEN BEANS, LIMA, LINTIL, RED BEANS, BLACK BEANS

BEVERAGES
WATER, SPARKLING WATER, UNSWEETEBD TEA

CARBS
BROWN-RICE, OAT-MEAL, POTATO, SWEET POTATO ALMONDS, WALNUTS, HAZELNUTS, MACADAMIA NUTS, PEANUTS, SUNFLOWER SEEDS, FLAXI SEEDS

FISH
BLUE FISH, CATFISH, COD, FLANK, FLOUNDER, FLUKE, HALIBUTT, RED SNAPPER, SEA BASS, TILAPIA, TROUT, TUNA, WHITTING.

POULTRY
CHICKEN-BREAST, TURKEY-BREAST, GROUND-TURKEY BREAST, GROUND-CHICKEN-BREAST.

VEGETABLES
BROCCOLI, BRUSSEL SPROUTS, CABBAGE, CARROTS, CAULIFLOWER, CUCUMBER, COLLARDS, CORN, CELERY, GINGER, GREEN PEPPER, GREEN PEAS, EGGPLANT, LETTUCE & ROMAINE, MUSHROOMS, OKRA, ONION, RADISH, RED PEPPER, SPINACH, STRING BEANS, SQUASH, TOMATO, YELLOW PEPPER

SPICES
APPLE CIDER-VINEGAR extra-virgin olive oil BAY-LEAF, CAYENNE PEPPER, CINNAMON, CUMIN, CURRY, DILL, GARLIC, MUSTARD, NUTMEG, ONION-POWDER, OREGANO, PAPRIKA, PARSLEY, PEPPER, SAGE, THYME, VINEGAR

SWEETNERS & miscellaneous
HONEY, SPLENDA UNSALTED RAW CASHEWS, RAW UNSALTED PENUTS EGG-BEATTERS. EGG WHITES

Oven baked Lemon Pepper Chicken

Ingredients

4 pieces of 6 0z. Boneless and skinless chicken breast

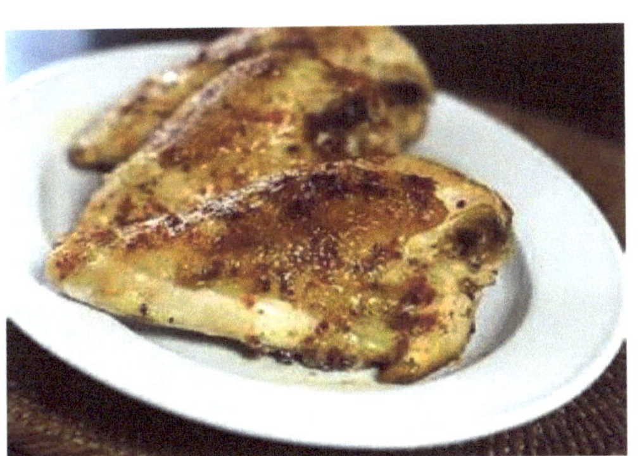

2 lemons

2 tsp. olive oil

2 tsp. minced garlic

1 tsp. sea Mrs. Dash

1 tsp. ground black pepper

1 tsp. onion powder

Instructions

Preheat the oven to 375 F. Cut the two lemons down the center and drain of all juices into a baking dish. Combine the olive oil, garlic, Mrs. Dash, pepper, and onion powder into the dish and blend. Wash off the pieces of chicken thoroughly. Then place in the marinade and turn the chicken over to coat on all sides. Bake for 20 minutes, then turn the chicken over and bake for an additional 10 minutes or until the chicken is

Cooked through.

Honey Glazed Chicken Breast

Ingredients

4-6 pieces of boneless and skinless chicken breast

4 tsp. extra-virgin olive oil

2 tsp. minced garlic

1/2-cup honey

1 tsp. lemon juice

1 tsp. chili powder

1 tsp. onion powder

1/2 tsp. garlic powder

1 lemon

Scallion stalk

Instructions

Wash off the pieces of chicken thoroughly. Then in a saucepan heat 1 tsp. of the olive oil set on medium heat. Add the minced garlic and stir until golden brown. Add the honey, chili powder garlic powder and onion powder then simmers for no more than a minute. Brush the chicken with the remaining 3 tablespoons olive then add to the sauce pan. Cover and let it cook for 15 minutes then turn over and cook for an additional 10 minutes or until chicken is thoroughly cooked. Slice the lemon and scallion stalk and use for decretive garnish.

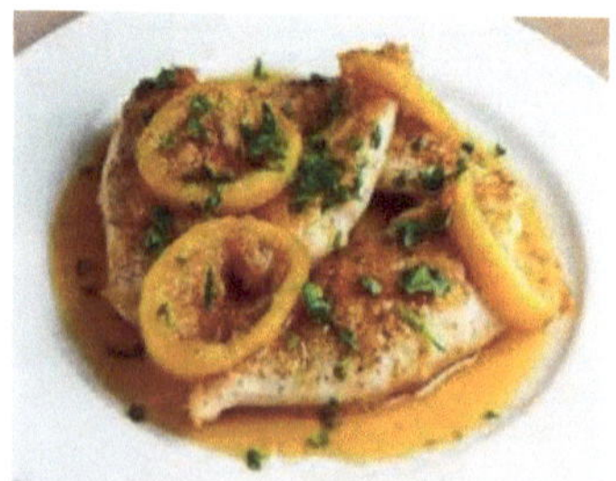

Seared Garlic Tilapia

Ingredients

Instructions

4 cloves garlic, finely diced

4 tablespoons olive oil

¼ tsp. Mrs. Dash

¼ tsp. garlic powder

1 tbs. chopped green pepper

In medium saucepan heat the olive oil then add the diced garlic and brown. Then remove the garlic and place in a bowl. Mix the Mrs. Dash, garlic powder together then rub it onto both sides of the fish. Begin to sauté the fish in the saucepan on both sides for 5 minutes or until thoroughly cooked. Quickly sauté green pepper in pan with non fat cooking spray then use for garnish.

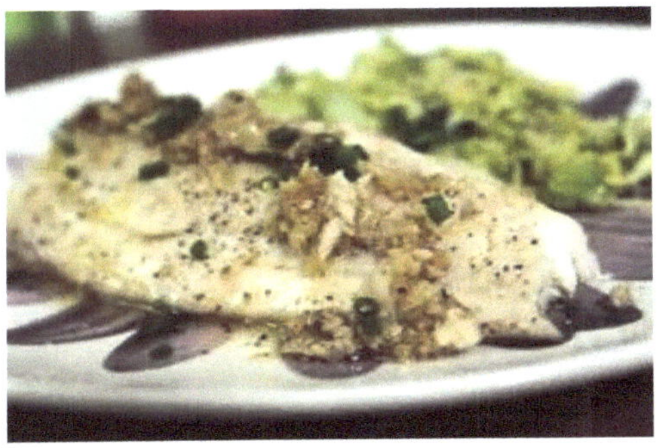

Garlic Olive Oil Flounder

Ingredients

1 pound fresh flounder fillets

2 tbs. olive oil

1 tablespoon chopped garlic

½ tsp. freshly ground black pepper

1 tsp. parsley

Pinch of ground pepper

Pinch Mrs. Dash

Slice lemon

Instructions

Wash off the pieces of fish thoroughly. Then preheat the oven to 350F. In a sauce bowl combine the olive oil. Garlic, pepper, parsley and sea-salt and mix for one minute. Lay out the pieces of fish in a baking pan and begin to brush the mixture onto both sides of the fish. Place in the oven and cook for 20 minute or until fish is thoroughly cooked. Then squeeze lemon juice over the fish when done and garnish with the remaining lemon.

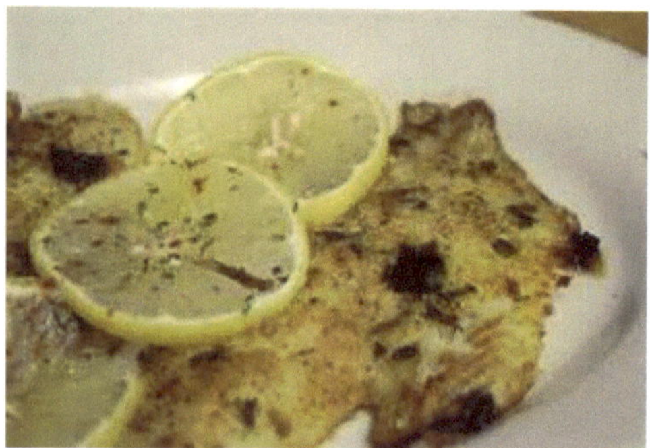

Chopped tomato Tilapia

Ingredients

2 (8-ounce) tilapia fillets

½ tsp. Mrs. Dash

½ tsp. ground black pepper

½ tsp. basil

½ tsp. oregano

1 tsp. onion powder

1 tsp. minced garlic

3 tablespoons olive oil

1 tsp. lemon juice

Dash of paprika

1 large tomato, chopped

Nonstick fat free cooking spray

Instructions

Wash off the pieces of fish thoroughly. Then preheat the oven to 350F. Spray baking pan with nonstick fat free cooking spray. In a medium bowl mix the olive oil, lemon juice, Mrs. Dash, pepper, basil, oregano, onion powder, garlic, and paprika. Brush the mixture evenly over the fish then place in the oven. Cook for 15 minutes then remove and cover the fish with the chopped tomato's then return to the oven for an additional 5 minutes or until thoroughly cooked.

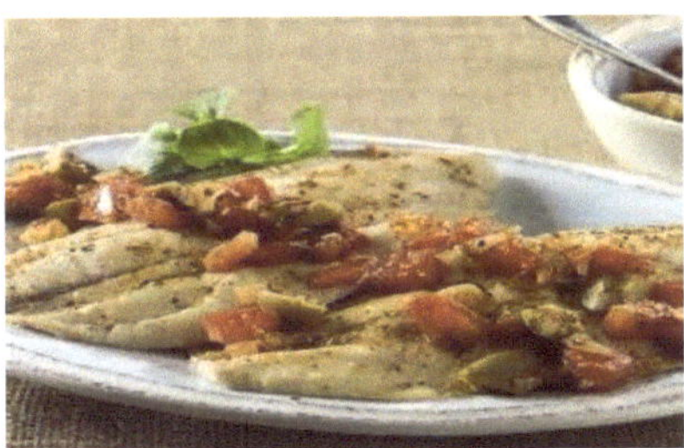

<h1 style="text-align:center">Baked Salmon Spinach Salad</h1>

Ingredients

1 salmon fillet 6 oz.

Pinch of Mrs. Dash

Pinch of paprika

½ tsp. garlic powder

1 tsp. olive oil

1 tsp. honey mustard

Non-stick fat free cooking spray

Instructions

Wash off the piece of fish thoroughly. Then preheat the oven to 400 F. Combine salt, paprika, garlic, olive oil, and mustard in a cup and mix. Spray baking pan with fat free cooking spray then place the salmon in center of the pan. Pour mixture over the fish evenly then place in the oven cook for 20 minutes or until fish flakes easily with a fork.

Salad

1-cup spinach   1 tsp. honey

1 tsp. olive oil   1 tsp. apple cider vinegar

Thoroughly rinse spinach then set aside on a plate. In a cup mix the olive oil, vinegar, honey. Pour the mixture over the spinach then set aside. Once the salmon is thoroughly cooked remove from pan and place it on top of the spinach and enjoy.

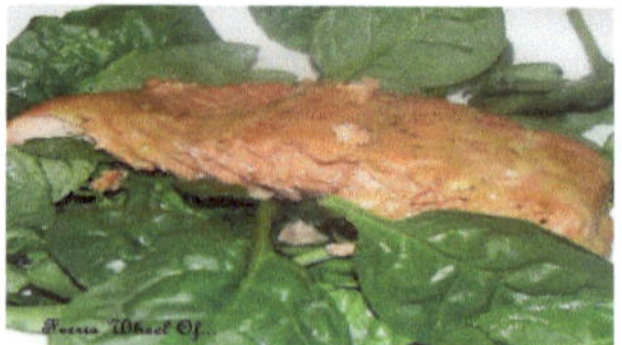

SAVORY BREAKFAST SAUSAGE

1) In a medium bowl, mix the following ingredients until well combined.
1lb of ground chicken or turkey breast.
2 tbsp. minced red onion
4 cloves garlic, minced
½ tsp. ground sage
½ tsp. dried thyme
½ tsp. cayenne pepper
½ tsp. fresh ground black pepper
Form the mixture into 11/2 inch-diameter meatballs. Flatten the balls to
Form patties about ¼ inches thick. Lightly coat the pan with non-fat
Cooking spray and set to medium-high until hot. Place the patties in the
Pan in a single layer (so they don't touch) and cook approximately 2-3
Minutes per side. Remove from pan when patties are no longer pink
Inside.

HASH BROWNS

Boil three small potatoes let cool then peel. Cut the potatoes in cubes,
Chop half a medium onion set aside. Take two cloves of garlic and chop
Cloves into small pieces and set aside. Wash and chop two green
Scallions. Cut one large green pepper in half the remove the seeds chop
And set aside. Coat the pan with non-fat cooking spray. Heat and sauté
Garlic, onions and green pepper for approximately 1 minute add
Potatoes to pan then season with.
½ Tspn. Curry powder
½ Tspn. Garlic powder
½ Tspn. Black pepper
½ Tspn. Thyme
When potatoes begin to brown turn heat to low and cook about 10
Minutes, stirring occasionally

BREAKFAST TURKEY HASH

1 Large (1 cup) red onion, diced ¼ inch..
3 Large red potatoes, diced ¼ inch.
1 Medium (1 cup) red bell pepper, diced ¼ inch.
1 Medium (1 cup) yellow bell pepper diced ¼ inch.
3 Cups turkey chopped
1 Teaspoon garlic salt.
1 Tablespoon black pepper
1 Egg white.

Chop turkey breast into pieces place in a bowl then add egg white mix
The turkey and egg white together and set aside. In a large skillet, over
Medium heat. Cook the onion in ¼ cup of water until brown. Add
Potatoes and continue to cook, stirring often for five minutes. Add
Peppers, seasoning and turkey. Cook until potatoes are soft and peppers
Are tender.

Potato curry chicken

8 oz chicken breast
2 medium potato's
½ medium onion
½ tsp. black pepper
½ tsp. garlic powder
½ tsp. thyme
1 tbsp. curry

First wash and cut chicken breast in 1inch cubes and set aside. Then
wash potatoes and prick all around with a fork. Boil until cooked cut
into ½ inch cuts. Then set aside. Peel and chop onions set aside. Then in
a standard frying pan spray with non-fat cooking spray and heat. Add
onions stir until brown then add chicken, potatoes, pepper, garlic, thyme
and curry. Cook on a low heat stir frequently allow to cook for 5min. Or
to your own taste.

LEMON PEPPER CHICKEN

8 oz Chicken breast
2 Medium fresh lemons
1 Medium egg (just the egg whites)
1 Tblsp. Pepper
½ Tsp. garlic powder

First preheat oven at 350, then wash chicken breast and set aside in a bowl. Then open one medium egg and separate the yoke. Place the egg white in the bowl with the chicken breast mix and set aside. Then press each lemon against the counter top with the palm of your hand, and roll against the counter top until soft. Cut each lemon in half and squeeze the juice over the breast, until the lemon is completely dry. Then add the pepper and garlic, place contents into a standard baking pan and bake for 25 to 30 minutes.

Sizzling red snapper

2 Slices of 4 to 8 oz red snapper
Garlic powder
Black pepper
Cayenne pepper
Curry powder
Chili powder
1 whole lime

Cut one whole lime in half and squeeze the juice from both half's of the lime completely over the fish. Then season both sides of the fish with garlic, black pepper, cayenne pepper, curry powder and chili powder to your taste. Bake fish in a preheated oven at 400 for about 12 to 15 minutes until it flakes apart.

During this program you should eat no less than four to six times a day. Follow the list, and remember if it is not on the list then you can not
eat it. You may place any combination together utilizing the list in any order or at any meal time.

DAILY MEAL PLAN EXAMPLES
Meal - 1 Savory breakfast sausage, hash browns.
Meal - 2 Potato curry chicken
Meal - 3 Garlic onion baked potato
Meal - 4 Sizzling red snapper
Meal - 5 Chicken salad
Meal - 6 Tuna salad

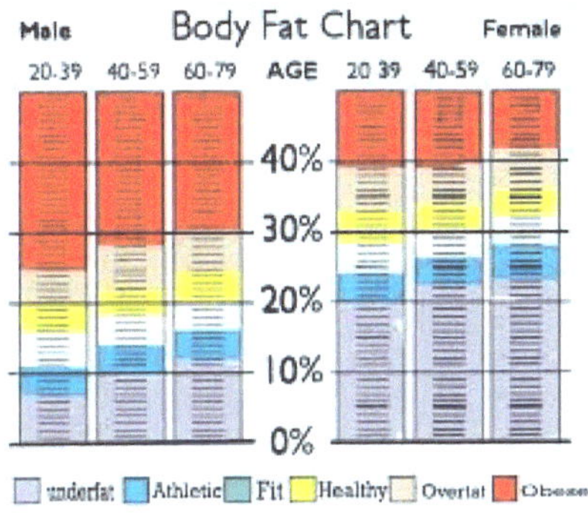

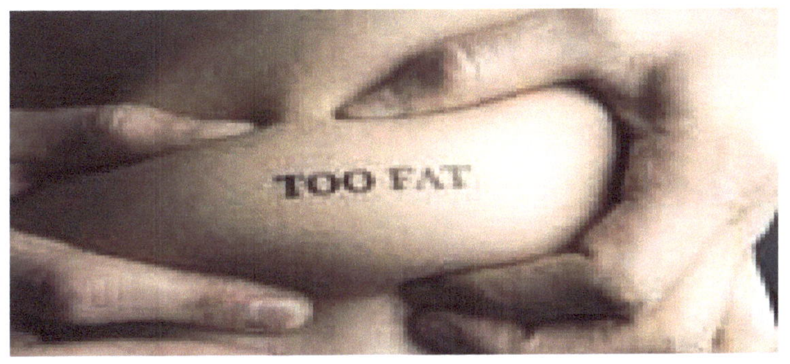

YOU MAY ALSO USE NON - FAT COOKING SPRAY IT'S THAT SIMPLE! EAT ANYTHING ON THE LIST. FOUR TO SIX TIMES A DAY, UTILIZE THE RECIPES IF YOU WISH. OR CREATE YOUR OWN RECIPES FROM ANYTHING ON THE LIST. THIS PROGRAM LAST ONLY THREE SHORT WEEKS AND YOU MAY CONTINUE FOR A LIFE TIME OF HEALTH AND GREAT NUTRITION.

REMEMBER IF IT IS NOT ON THE LIST, THEN NO! YOU CAN NOT EAT IT!

View your list, these are the foods that can be eaten during this program.